PROSTATE RECOVERY MAP

3rd Ed.

Men's Action Plan

T0348143

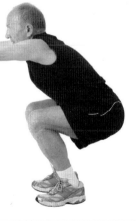

A/Prof. CRAIG ALLINGHAM

Prostate Recovery MAP

Published by Redsok International
PO Box 1881, Buderim, Qld. Australia. 4556
Office 3.05, 1 Kings Street, London, UK, EC2V 8AU

2013, 2014 (revised & updated)
2nd Edition 2017
3rd Edition 2020, 2022
www.redsok.com

National Library of Australia Cataloguing-in-Publication entry

Author: Allingham, Craig

Title: Prostate Recovery MAP: Men's Action Plan / Craig Allingham

ISBN: **978-0-9870766-8-7**

Subjects: Urinary incontinence   Dewey Number: 616.62

Prostate--Diseases--Patients--Popular works
Prostate--Cancer--Patients--Popular works
Generative organs, Male--Diseases--Popular works
Impotence--Popular works
Bladder--Popular works

Images on pages 17, 37, 41, 52 sourced and acknowledged from Wikimedia Commons

Printed in Australia by InkSpot Printers, Maroochydore, Qld.

2

MAP Contents

Dedication

*To my father, Gordon Allingham, who taught me much
and loved me more.*

Acknowledgements

I am very grateful to all who have assisted with the ongoing development, content and evolution of Men's Action Plan.

Advice: Peter Dornan, Stuart Doobar-Baptist, Dr. Jo Milios & Dr. Beth Shelly

Reviewers: Dr Michael Gillman & Fiona Rogers

Mary O'Dwyer author and teacher for women's health who pointed out that 'men need information too.'

From the Author

My personal reason for writing this book has not changed since the first edition in 2013. My Dad had prostate cancer and spent years undergoing various treatments initially to cure him, and later to extend his quality of life. He was one of many pioneers for prostate cancer treatment providing outcome data for doctors and patients yet to come. His illness and the challenges he faced prompted my interest in men's health and my professional conversion from elite sports physiotherapy to men recovering from prostate treatment.

The updated second edition (2017) included several changes in prostate disease management and recovery. New exercises for continence and erectile function enhanced the MAP program.

This third edition follows the release of my Prostate Playbook in 2019, which provides information and strategies for reducing prostate cancer onset, progression and recurrence. Some of this new material is referenced or updated in this book.

Recent research in men with prostate cancer suggests the mental burden can be as incapacitating as the physical side-effects of treatment. Depression and reduced quality of life have many men experiencing 'decision regret'. This book provides a positive, practical and evidence based program to help men take control of their own outcomes - to claim back some mastery as they navigate, adapt to and accept their new reality.

Every man who applies himself will show some improvement. The MAP rewards effort and persistence and some of you may lose heart or interest before seeng the benefits. You may need to revisit this book when you feel overwhelmed, exhausted and vulnerable. All the best.

Craig Allingham APAM, FSMA

B.App.Sc.(Physio), Grad.Dip.Sport Sci., Cert. Men's Hlth., Exec.MBA.
Adjunct A/Prof Bond University Faculty of Health, Science & Medicine

Unfolding the MAP

This section provides an introduction to the elements of the updated Men's Action Plan (MAP). You will see how they piece together and follow a logical sequence from basic to complex, from light to heavy, from slow to fast and from wet to dry. Each level has a purpose and rates of progress will vary. Some levels will prove easy while others may take weeks or months to master. Be patient.

Any procedure that messes with the prostate has the potential to disturb your waterworks and erectile function. The minor procedures done via the penis/urethra (resections, rebores, etc.) rarely cause long term issues. Serious surgery involving removal of the prostate gland either by a radical open, laparascopic or robotic procedure is more likely to challenge your bladder control.

You will not find information or guidance for deciding what prostate treatment (if any) is right for you. You need to discuss your specific case with your medical provider and/or urologist. There are many variables in prostate disease: your family history, age and medical condition, which are further compounded by the medical test results (PSA, Gleason Scores, biopsy, MRI and PET scans) all of which make general treatment recommendations not only unwise but inappropriate.

Here is an overview:

Before Surgery: Learn how to do the pelvic floor training effectively. Try and get at least four weeks training for surgery. In addition to the training, this is a great time to review other lifestyle factors impacting on your long term recovery and health outcomes. For example food and fluid intake, physical activity patterns and quality and quantity of sleep. By the way, research shows it is better to be taught how to do exercises by a professional rather than learn them from a paper handout or from the internet. If you find elements of the MAP program unclear I have uploaded videos to YouTube to help out (p.60). If still not sure, take this book along to your health provider and seek clarification.

This pre-operative time is valuable yet often under-utilised. Many guys put more preparation into purchasing an audio system or a new car than they do into preparing themselves for important surgery and the follow up. Don't be too cool or heroic to take this seriously. Do your research, seek and listen to advice then commit to the program early. This will give you the best chance of a great outcome.

Research suggests the best chance of having erectile function following prostate surgery is to have good function pre-surgery. Try and get some practice in, or work with some medication. Check out page 51. Was that discrete enough?

After Surgery: While the urinary catheter is in place (tube in penis, bag on leg) don't resume the pelvic floor exercises. Focus on resting, good nutrition and gently resuming activity levels. Once the catheter is removed, restart at Level One of the MAP.

- » **Level One** - mastering technique and endurance training for your pelvic floor muscles
- » **Level Two** - power training to control leaking under load
- » **Level Three** - bladder training to increase volume and time between emptying
- » **Level Four** - integration of your pelvic floor expertise into other daily activities and exercises
- » **Level Five** - masterclass training for the unexpected
- » **Level Six** - reducing risk of recurrence

The first five levels are discussed in the following pages. Level Six leads on to The Prostate Playbook (see page 64). Short YouTube videos are available at www.craigallingham.com.

Radiation Treatment: this is less problematic in terms of continence at least in the short term. It is still worth learning and training the exercises to ensure you are starting out as pelvic-fit as possible.

Long After Treatment: We are talking about muscle training and skills so your improvement will be maintained only for as long as you continue to train. The maintenance training is less demanding, but it is vital for your ongoing success. All going well you will have many years of pelvic floor training ahead. Age related changes may impact on your continence, and meanwhile you will have stopped the training once happy with your results. If you have any deterioration (leaking, erectile, urgency, frequency, after-wee) revisit this book. Don't pass it on to a mate - tell him where to get his own copy. Things change, and resuming the training may slow or reverse any losses.

It is not reading the Men's Action Plan that makes the difference, it is completing the training. Your success depends on you negotiating the exercises, self tests, training progressions and the new mind set of post-cancer survivorship.

You don't have to do this alone. Seek and accept help from your life partner, family, medical support team, physiotherapist, local support group, and various other resources and agencies that can help. Some of us prefer to be a solo traveller, and for you this book will be even more useful.

<u>You</u> are in charge of the MAP

Be the leader, ask questions, read stuff, discuss with your support team and listen to advice. It is your responsibility to find your way, keep on going and take control. That's what men can do.

Welcome To My World

Here is the typical story I hear in my clinic, it might not be your exact story but some elements may sound familiar.

Craig: So Bob, tell me what has been happening in your life recently?

Bob: Well, Prof, a few months back my doctor found an lump on my prostrate* and my PSA had shot up in the last few months.

Craig: Excuse me Bob, but it is called a prostate, and what was your PSA?

Bob's Wife: It was more than a few months ago, it was last year and I told you to get checked sooner. And now look at you.

Bob: I'm not sure, above 5 I think. Well anyway, after more tests..

Craig: A biopsy? MRI?

Bob: Yeah, a biopsy, they found a cancer on the prostrate* and it had to come out.

Craig: Prostate. When was that done, mate, and how has it turned out?

Bob's Wife: It went great, we are now cancer free.....

Craig: Bob?

Bob: The Doc said the surgery went well and he got it all. Which was a great relief, but...

Craig: That is great news, and have you had the PSA follow up?

Bob: Not yet, in a few months.

---

*No. PROSTATE - only one 'r'. More on page 12.

Craig: So how did things go after surgery in terms of the waterworks?

Bob's Wife: He is still having lots of problems. Can't go without pads and...

Bob: Yeah, I am still having problems which is why the Doc sent me to you. After the surgery when they took the catheter out I just ran like a tap and I was pretty worried. This settled down over a couple of days and I thought it would gradually sort itself out, but it stopped improving and now I have to wear pads all the time.

Craig: How do you feel about that?

Bob: I hate them. They are uncomfortable, they smell.

Bob's Wife: Not as much as you think.

Bob: And I don't really trust them, so I don't go out much in case I have an accident. And I look weird with my new shoulder bag.

Craig: What is happening with your work?

Bob: I run a building firm and I have blokes doing the jobs at the moment, but I will need to get back into it to drum up work and to keep things running. Trouble is, I don't want them to see me like this.... I didn't think it would be so bad. Every time I stand up, or cough or bend over I squirt. And there seems to be a constant slow drip that I can't even feel, but the pads get wetter. I go through two or three pads most days and another one at night, more if I have a beer. I feel OK and am happy the cancer is gone, but I.... this leaking is..... I can't.... it's ruining my life. Can you help me?

Summary

Bob's wife is concerned. Bob is a bit down, maybe even depressed. The extent of his urine leaking is unexpected and interfering with his life and planned return to work. He is disappointed and confused. He sought advice, made a decision to have surgery and followed all the instructions afterwards. Why is he not getting better? Why wasn't he told how bad this leaking could be? If he had known, would he have followed a different path?

Bob's story is very familiar to me, including his helpful wife. In hindsight, would Bob have followed a different path? Probably not. The desire to remove the cancer from his body before it spreads to other more critical body parts (perhaps becoming life shortening) is very powerful and the impact of incontinence and erectile dysfunction are not fully appreciated despite being discussed with the doctor and in the patient literature. After all, what is some leaking compared with a cancer that may or may not spread? And Bob's wife is a powerful presence: a stakeholder in his outcomes and a partner in their journey. Her fears for him are about survival not continence. And regarding the erection issue, who is going to know apart from Bob and his wife? Better to live a soft life than be stiff all over. (Sorry, too soon?)

Can I help him? Yes, definitely. Can I 'cure' his incontinence? Too early to say. I need to find out more of Bob's history, his lifestyle factors, if he did any pre-operative exercise program, what (if any) exercises he has been doing since surgery and test him to see if he is performing them correctly. My experience shows an active pelvic floor training program will reduce Bob's leakage to some extent, and most often to the point of no longer needing to wear pads. He has nothing to lose and lots to gain.

All or part of Bob's story may apply to you, and the difference between him and you is obvious: I can't physically examine you to identify your muscle performance, timing, strength, endurance and control.

What I recommend specifically for Bob may not be appropriate for you or ten other men. However, in my experience, there are sufficient shared factors to present a program covering the common issues and offering likely solutions. Some of the material in this book will work for you, some might not, but none of it will harm or slow your recovery.

When considering the material in this book remember you may also need some individual guidance from your medical support team. The information, tests and activities contained here may get you some or all of the way. **Doing nothing will change nothing.**

A men's health or continence physiotherapist will be able check how well you are performing your exercises, reassure you, correct you and determine the best daily exercise routine to suit your stage of recovery or pattern of incontinence. Some may use imaging technology (real time ultrasound) to help you better understand and perform the exercises in this book. Not all physiotherapists are trained in this area of men's health. You may have to actively seek the right practitioner by asking your doctor or surgeon or on the website of the national association where you can often search practitioners based on the services they offer. A local prostate cancer support group will also know the nearby services on offer.

On Pronunciation

As a health professional, when Bob mispronounces his disease it concerns me. I subconsciously wonder how much attention he is really giving to his problem? Is he hearing the information and advice offered? Is he taking this serious matter seriously. If he can't get the word right, how will he go with the exercises, nutrition and activity demands? After all, Bob wouldn't mispronounce something important like his preferred fishing tackle, his favourite exotic car or the names of his children. This is important too.

It's A Design Thing

The prostate gland is a mix of muscle and gland tissue and is wrapped around your urethra (the tube carrying urine from bladder to the penis). This urethra is a soft tube, pliable and collapsible. When you pinch your penis to stop urine flow you are collapsing the urethra and blocking flow. When the muscles around the urethra are contracted, they also collapse the tube and prevent leakage. The prostate muscles are really good at this which is a design advantage because when you are squirting seminal fluid out from the prostate (ejaculating) these muscles are simultaneously blocking the urethra behind to prevent urine release and propel the sperm along the southern route.

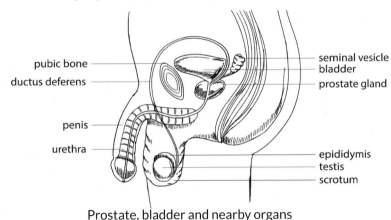

Prostate, bladder and nearby organs

With the urethra passing through the prostate, any enlargement, swelling, tumour growth or inflammation of the gland can compromise your waterworks function. Symptoms of prostate disease include frequency of toilet calls, difficulty initiating flow, a weak or split urine stream and after-dribble.

In benign growths of the prostate (enlargement), a surgical procedure is performed through the urethra itself[*] to stretch the collapsed area or to cut away the intruding prostate tissue to decompress the tube and regain good urine flow.

When a prostate cancer is removed surgically, the prostate tissue must be cut away from the urethra which can be very difficult, especially if the cancer margins are not clear. It is likely that the segment of the urethra within the prostate will be taken by the surgeon and the free end on the penis side reattached to the base of the bladder. A recent study indicates around 4% of men felt that their penis was shorter after prostate removal. This is due to altered nerve input, loss of elasticity from 'disuse' and/or loss of urethral length. Four in one hundred is a small number, and may well be under-reported, but if you are one of them it is just another slap in the face. This outcome is difficult to predict before surgery as it depends on the cancer complexity, the skill of the surgeon, your general health and your post-op erectile training (see penile rehabilitation p. 51).

When the prostate is removed, so is the muscle within the gland which has been helping with urine flow regulation. Because the intra-prostate muscle is not under voluntary control, there is no way of knowing how much use each bloke makes of it in helping to control urine flow. Some men may use it a lot, others not at all, which is alright because there are other muscles at the base of the bladder that also seal the flow. However, if you were a prostate-muscle-user all your life and that muscle has been removed, it may take a while to find and train the bladder and pelvic floor muscle back-up system after surgery.

This is why I strongly recommend starting your bladder control program (pelvic floor exercises) prior to surgery, making sure all relevant muscle systems are engaged and ready for the upcoming challenges. Six weeks beforehand is a good time to start and certainly no less than four weeks. Establishing this

---

14   *Known as 'pee-hole surgery'. Not really, but it should be. Opportunity lost.*

exercise habit is difficult and important. Difficult because there is no apparent need (yet) to do them; and important because a regular habit of exercising will be easier to resume after surgery than to commence for the first time. There are other difficulties ahead without adding laziness to the list.

Four weeks or so before you are due to undergo prostate surgery or radiotherapy I recommend you learn and train daily on the Level One exercises (see page 20). You may be tempted to go beyond to other levels, I like your enthusiasm, but be sure to master the Level One techniques which is where you will recommence the program after treatment.

A study from the Westmead Hospital in Sydney established that men who underwent physiotherapy guided pelvic floor muscle training for four weeks prior to surgery experienced a significant improvement in the duration and severity of their early incontinence following their radical prostatectomy[1]. Meaning, if you want faster improvement after surgery, get stuck into this program at least four weeks beforehand. Now you know.

Other research suggests erectile recovery is more likely for those men who had satisfactory erectile function pre-surgery, so if you are out of condition (so to speak), try to exercise your erectile function before the surgery. Sounds easy, but you will likely be in a state of some anxiety regarding your diagnosis and confusion around treatment decisions, work arrangements, financial matters and so on. Not the optimal circumstances for romance. Talk with your partner, acknowledge the challenges and find a way to work together on some erectile stimulation. Or you may need to go solo. This is erectile training, not ejaculation or penetration - they are optional extras. Twice per week should be sufficient training but if you can manage more, why not?

---

1. Yao J, Hirschhorn A, Mungovan S, Patel M. 2012. Preoperative pelvic floor physiotherapy improves continence following radical prostatectomy. J Neurourology & Urodynamics, 31(6):964

Why Might It Be Difficult?

The guys I see in the clinic following their prostate surgery are those who are not doing very well or are unsure of what exercises to do and how they should be done. The men who sail through with rapid recovery of bladder control are not my clients. I may have worked with them before surgery but not afterwards and phone follow-up confirms this MAP has contributed to their success.

There are several factors working **short term** against regaining your bladder control. They include:

> » You have had major surgery around your plumbing, including a reattached urethra. Things have been pushed and pulled about a bit, nerves stretched and arteries cauterized. It hurts and may still be bleeding - which will show in your urine. The first week or so can be uncomfortable and provides no reliable guide as to how you will go after the catheter is removed.

> » The catheter holds the bladder mouth open and stretches the muscle sphincter that will later have to seal the opening to the urethra. Often, removal of the catheter is accompanied by ongoing, unstoppable and distressing urine flow. It may take up to a day or so for the stretched sphincter muscle to regain tone. Guys find this unstoppable urine flow very upsetting and fear the surgery has gone wrong and they will need to wear the catheter for the rest of their lives. But they don't voice this concern or ask anyone, they just worry. This does not help. Use the pads until it resolves.

> » Pain. Post-surgical pain can interfere with muscle control. Make sure you have adequate pain management with

the help of your doctor. None of the exercises should cause pain in or around the operation site or elsewhere (e.g. lower back). If they do, discontinue and consult a physiotherapist or other health professional.

These three factors will resolve with time and many guys regain most bladder control within a few weeks of removal of the catheter. These men were probably not prostate-muscle users during their lives, and their preferred muscles were still in place and relearning their job.

Beyond these short term factors there are further issues that can prevent or delay regaining bladder control in the **longer term**:

» Nerve damage during surgery. Your surgeon will strive to carefully separate the prostate gland from the surrounding nerves and blood vessels before resecting (cutting) the gland free. However the gland is enclosed in a fibrous mesh and separation is often challenging and may cause collateral damage in terms of cutting of nerves (permanent damage) or stretching of nerves as they are dissected away (temporary damage at least).

» Poor bladder control before surgery. If you have leakage issues before the operation the likelihood of ongoing problems afterwards is higher. This is another good argument for beginning the program before surgery.

» Obesity. The greater the weight resting down on your bladder from above the more pressure and load leading to leaking. This is simple physics: add gravity and an upright position and the only way is down. A big gut is a bladder squeezer. More at page 38.

» Generic exercise instruction. Standard procedure in many hospitals is for a continence nurse or a physiotherapist to visit you after surgery and instruct you in your pelvic floor muscle exercises. Generally these professionals give you a brief period of instruction, leave a couple of leaflets behind and wish you all the best. One recent client of mine was given two different handouts which contradicted each other! It was like having two conflicting maps and trying to work out which way to go. He was very confused.

Research evidence on learning an exercise (a skill) shows the outcome from a written handout is inferior to an instructional session from someone expert at teaching the skill. I have proved this by trying to play golf from a book (badly) and then improving with the same information, immediate feedback and correction from a golf pro. My poor golf is now solely due to a lack of practice.

» Failing to follow instructions. Seriously? A man not following instructions? Many guys are experts in other areas of their lives and for some reason believe they are now experts in recovering from prostate surgery or have a misguided faith in their powers of recovery. Perhaps they didn't quite get the proper picture in the first place as to how much of their recovery was going to be up to their personal contribution. Then there is the laziness option.

» Bad luck. Yep, surgical complications; incomplete resection of the gland, infections, scar tissue blocking the reattached urethra and so on. Not all of these procedures go smoothly. There is always risk and your surgeon is duty bound to tell you about them. Pay attention, ask questions and there will be fewer surprises.

When you discover a cancer in your body all your resolve is focused on removing the threat. Once removed, the very real complications you were warned of become apparent. They are now your most important issue because the cancer has been dealt with. Leaking urine and erectile dysfunction were previously insignificant and intangible against the cancer threat. Now they are real and impacting on your quality of life. I have had several clients comment sadly 'If I knew how bad the incontinence would be, I wouldn't have had the op'. However on an individual level we can never know beforehand.

Pad Up! Pad Up! And Play the Game! *

A percentage of men who undergo prostate surgery do not become fully continent. Their daily life involves ongoing use of continence pants, pads, tissues or urine collectors (e.g. Urox). For some this is an intolerable inconvenience and embarrassment. For others it is a means to continue being active and involved with work, family, social and recreational pursuits. The second group is much happier.

If, having given the Men's Action Plan a serious go, consulted continence professionals and attended support groups, you still need to use pads here is my advice to you:

PAD UP

TUCK IN

PLAY ON

Life can still be good, much better than it may have been otherwise. If wearing a garment or pads is all you have to worry about - get over it - there is plenty of life you can still enjoy. How much will be entirely up to you. Don't be a victim, be a master. You are not in a battle, you are delivering a project.

Alternatively, you could discuss with your urologist any advances in surgical techniques including artificial sphincters or support slings that may be appropriate for your situation.

With apologies to Sir Henry Newbolt, English Poet, 1862-1938. This is an adaption of the line 'Play up! play up! and play the game!' from his poem 'Vitaï Lampada' meaning 'the torch of life'. Quite appropriate, really.

Level One - Mastery Starts Here

Mastering control of your bladder storage and release is not just a matter of exercising muscles, it is far more complex. Just as serving a tennis ball is not simply a matter of toss and hit (it involves strategy, subterfuge, timing and cunning <u>plus</u> toss and hit), your pelvic floor muscle retraining will also involve many layers of skill development, concentration and focus.

Being men, once we hear the words 'muscle' and 'exercise' we figure the harder we go the better and quicker the results will be. The most common error I see in the clinic is guys going at the exercises too hard. The second most common error is exercising the wrong muscles. Both groups of guys are very good at *their* version of the exercises. It is a pity they are very good at doing them wrongly, thereby getting better and better at being worse. In fact some are actually training themselves to leak more, rather than less.

In this Men's Action Plan you are not just exercising muscles to regain continence, you are learning to master a skill. It is a skill you have had since graduating from toilet training and have never thought much about except after a dodgy oyster, a powerful curry or too much light beer (which I find is far more testing for the bladder than the full strength version). MAP is a **skill-based** program and in Level One there are three critical elements:

>   » Correct Muscles
>   » Correct Technique
>   » Correct Prescription

Correct Muscles

Front ones, not the back ones. It is more important to lift your testicles than to stop a fart. They are both important, but in terms of your bladder control the front muscles of your pelvic floor must be activated to improve continence. These pelvic floor muscles are under voluntary control and when you activate them they constrict and kink the urethra below the bladder connection reducing flow-through. These are the muscles you would activate to interrupt your urine flow mid-stream at the toilet. That is the sensation you are trying to reproduce.

SELF TEST:

Stand up. Strip down so you can see your belly and imagine you are interrupting urine flow midstream (no hands). Watch your lower abdominal wall - if it moves inwards more than just slightly you are over-trying. Your testicle-lifting, urine-interrupting muscles will not flatten your belly. However if you try too hard and suck in your navel in an attempt to stop flow you are now recruiting your deep abdominal muscles. When these contract they increase intra-abdominal pressure compressing the bladder and making it more difficult to interrupt flow. If your abs are working more than your pelvic floor muscles you may leak during or immediately after the exercise AND you will become extremely proficient at squeezing your bladder. Not useful.

If you can feel a sensation of lifting the testicles or a shortening of the penis WITH NO MOVEMENT of the abdominal wall - fantastic you are using the right muscles. Mind you, we don't need to tell anyone about this short penis and high testicle business.

Correct Technique

There are two ways to check this. One involves a rubber glove and one doesn't. Leave the glove version to me but try this one at home. Pants down and place one of your fingers immediately behind your scrotum (ball sack) and in front of your anus. Push up and you will feel it is squishy, keep some pressure on the area and repeat the self test described above. If you get it right you should feel a very slight firming of the squishy tissue as the muscle contracts. You might need to move a little off centre and try forward and back to find the muscle but when you do, the firming should correlate with your efforts at lifting your testicles and/ or shortening your penis. You should feel the muscle switch on (firm) and switch off (squishy). Switching off is just as important as switching on. Let it go.

Not only is this a gentle exercise, it is also a really slow one. The correct technique is a slow ramping activation, like turning up the volume rather than flicking a switch. Imagine you are turning up the volume steadily then holding for up to ten seconds. Don't turn the volume up to maximum, not yet anyway. Turn the volume (muscle activation) up to around 30% of maximum. This should reduce the abdominal muscle over-ride. If 30% intensity is possible with no abdominal activation, you can try for 40%, all the time checking on the ab muscle situation. Forty percent is the upper limit for this slow ramping exercise. When you release after ten seconds you should feel the unfirming back to squishy. If not, you probably faded out trying to hold beyond your limit. Next time try holding for only eight seconds, or six until you are certain of feeling the switch-off as you relax. This is now your duration of hold-time when training.

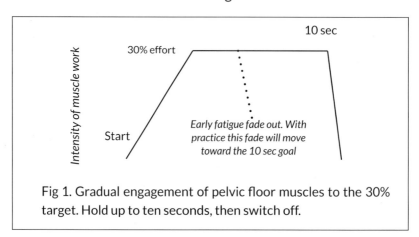

Fig 1. Gradual engagement of pelvic floor muscles to the 30% target. Hold up to ten seconds, then switch off.

Don't be concerned if you can't feel this easily yet. There is some fatty tissue in the way and/or you may not be getting the muscle activating enough to feel it firm. I recommend guys do this in the shower where there is no clothing barrier, some privacy and it doesn't seem so weird*. Of course, if he can't feel it firming, a sensible man will try harder and harder until he uses his abdominal muscles to suck in and up - once again tricking himself by trying too hard. Correct technique is more important than brute force, as it is for many things.

Belly Flop - to combat the urge to flatten or suck in your abdominal wall, simply do the opposite - gently bulge outwards and let it relax there. Flop that belly while maintaining a tall posture, with your chest up and head raised. Flop your belly in isolation - don't flop your entire posture into a slump.

When you do this exercise in standing, your bladder is weighing down on your pelvic floor muscles. As you activate them, you are trying to lift a little and initially may not have the strength to lift the bladder and its contents. I teach this exercise in a side-lying position to take gravity out of the picture. Lie on one side with both knees bent up a little toward your chest (sound familiar?). Reach down to the perineum area (behind the ball sack, in front of the anus) and do the exercise as described. When you get confident about your technique you can try it in standing, knees slightly bent and chest raised so your posture is tall. Now lift those testicles. Shorten that penis! Relax your butt & abs.

Breathing. It appears to be human nature to hold your breath whilst you are trying to lift your testicles or draw your penis back into your body. Who would have thought? However, unless you only want to have bladder control while holding your breath you will need to train yourself to hold the muscle tension below while

---

If you still think it is weird, try being in one of my workshops where up to twenty men are all feeling behind their scrotums and staring at the floor to avoid eye contact with any and every man in the room.

breathing normally. This is not as easy as it first appears. Your diaphragm muscle gently moves down as you breathe in and up as you breathe out. The diaphragm forms the roof of your abdominal cavity and because it is a closed space, when this roof moves down (breathing in) the floor muscles you are trying to activate and lift slightly are under extra load. You really will have to concentrate to master this aspect of the skill.

To reduce the tendency to hold your breath, follow your breathing as you prepare to tense your pelvic floor and initiate the lift during the out-breath. Then continue to breathe normally while sustaining the muscle tension down below.

Correct Prescription

Chances are your pelvic floor muscles are very weak and under-trained. It will not take many repetitions to fatigue them and once fatigued you will automatically seek out nearby abdominal and rectal muscles in an effort to sustain the tension. You should only continue the exercise for as long as you are certain the right muscles are still doing the job. If you lose the sensation internally or beneath your finger pressure, your exercise session is done for now. Note how many successful repetitions (reps) you have completed and make this your training prescription for now. The rate of fatigue will also depend on the duration of hold time. To limit the number of variables, let's make this a five second hold time and count the reps to fatigue. Fatigue may show as a loss of sensation (as above) or the initiation of the abdominal flattening as a compensation strategy. When you can do ten confident holds for the five seconds, you start to extend the hold time towards the ten second goal.

How many is enough? Fair question; if you fatigue quickly you will need to do more sessions per day, each one to your fatigue level. My suggested target is 60 *good repetitions* per day. So if you can do six reps to fatigue, you will need to do ten sets per day. If you can do 15 reps, you only need do four sets per day. Sixty 'good' repetitions per day: a good repetition is one you are certain used the right muscles with the right technique. If not, it doesn't count in the 60 reps. So concentrate, and get them right so you can get them done. Sixty reps, each for five seconds is only 300 seconds or five minutes of work over 24 hours. Even you can find that. To get used to working against gravity, do 20 reps in the side lying position, 20 in sitting and 20 in standing - do this every day and only count the good ones.

Your target for Level One is to complete sixty ten-second holds every day for a week with each set comprising at least ten repetitions. This may take three weeks or three months with persistent training depending on your starting point and consistency of application.

Problem Solving

Transition to Standing - a lot of blokes can do this exercise really well lying down, but have trouble feeling any activity in standing. It is a lot harder to execute upwards against the weight of the bladder and other organs pressing down. Try the following strategies:

» Spend another few days or a week just getting the 60 contractions done in a position you can definitely feel it working. It might be 30/30 lying down and sitting or the whole 60 lying on the bed or floor. Be patient but persistent. Every couple of days try the standing version until you detect activity.

» Supported Standing Position (SSP): stand at a bench or table with your hands on the surface. Support your upper body weight by leaning forward onto your hands whilst you bend your knees slightly. Keep your chest lifted and head raised, don't collapse your torso onto your hands. Now try the standing exercise again: take a deep breath in then as you slowly release the breath, gently and slowly raise your pelvic floor.

Expectation

You should improve at doing the exercise within a few days and after a week should start to see slight improvement in terms of leakage (less) and duration between peeing (longer) and stream quality (stronger). After two weeks of consistent work (60 good ones per day) you will be impressed with the improvement and extending your ability to hold longer during each rep. If not, consult your health professional again.

Summary of Level One

» Use the front-lifting, stream-interrupting muscles - feel with your fingers to detect their activity.

» Gentle and slow - you are not lifting weights with this thing.

» Do the Belly Flop, tall posture and breathe normally

» Sixty per day - concentrate, vary position and only count the good ones.

» Extend the hold-time as it becomes easier.

CAN'T FEEL THE SWITCHING OFF?

Not all men have a weak or inactive pelvic floor. Some have a pelvic floor that is constantly switched on and unable to fully relax or lengthen. This can lead to pelvic pain, an inability to empty the bladder and/or constipation.

For these men, the ability to relax and lengthen their pelvic floor muscles must be learned before any activation and strengthening exercises. A program of 'down-training' involving stretching and conscious relaxation strategies will need professional instruction as it goes against your natural urge to hold on.

If you can't feel the switch-off phase or the MAP exercises seem to be making you worse - stop. You must consult a pelvic floor physiotherapist for a program to suit your current challenge. You can resume the MAP program later.

Level Two - Bring the Power

Well done on mastering Level One - you are confidently using the right muscles, with the correct technique and have achieved a week or so at the training dose of 60 quality reps per day. If not, how can you be certain you are ready to move on to Level Two? Let's check:

SELF TESTING

1. Standing. Perform ten 50% intensity, slow contractions of the correct muscles without flattening your abs and with a clear sensation of both the turning on and turning off and a hold time of 10 seconds each. Count how many you can complete up to a maximum of ten.

2. Standing. Perform one maximal pelvic floor contraction holding to exhaustion or 60 seconds, whichever comes first.*

If you can complete 8-10 of the first test and at least 30 seconds of the second test you are ready to progress to Level Two. If not, keep training for another week or so and test again. It is important to meet the goals of Level One in order to maximise your gains at all of the following levels.

Ready to go? Excellent. So far you have been training the slow-twitch muscles fibres in your pelvic floor. These are the high endurance, low power and low speed fibres that provide sustained holding control of your full bladder against the downward load when you are up and about. These are the fibres that give you confidence to leave the house, or to wait a bit longer before you empty, and result in less pad use (and considerable savings).

However, they provide little protection against higher loads like coughing, laughing, sneezing, getting up from a chair, fast

* *Thanks to Dr Jo Milios, a Perth-based colleague, for her research on this Sustained Endurance Test.*

movement of your body or landing down off a step. They fail on these activities because they are slow activators. Level Two exercises will start training your fast-activating muscle fibres to provide rapid control when needed.

Now for the good news - it is not a new exercise. Same muscles but different intensity and two new patterns of activation.

Fire & Hold

Fast-switch will be important when you are upright and active, so you train in sitting or standing position. Focus, relax abs and butt, now <u>instantly</u> turn on the pelvic floor muscles to your maximum then promptly ease back to your familiar 30% range. Now hold, and hold..... hold for ten seconds or more if you can. This feels different to the dimmer-switch exercise you have been doing. Now you activate immediately, like a flick-switch (instant ON). These fast-twitch fibres are good at switching on but lousy at holding and they will fade away within a few seconds. To achieve the hold phase you will need to ease back to a lower intensity (Fig.2). Your explosive start activates the fast-twitch fibres, the lower level hold sustains the slow-twitch fibres meaning both power and endurance receive a training stimulus.

The muscle fibres are 'fast-twitch', and your exercise is 'fast-switch'. One is a type of muscle fibre, the other is the speed of your exercise initiation.

If you are fatiguing during the hold phase, take a second grab and get back to the 30% intensity. As you progress, this fatigue point will take longer to arrive until you find you can go the distance. But only if you train.

You may find the intensity of your 'fire' starts to fatigue after several repetitions and you can't feel the same intensity of switching on, but you still feel the second grab. It is likely that the fast-twitch (low endurance) fibres will fatigue first and you lose the ability to instantly flick-on. When this happens, the exercise is done. Your fast fibres are exhausted and will take some minutes

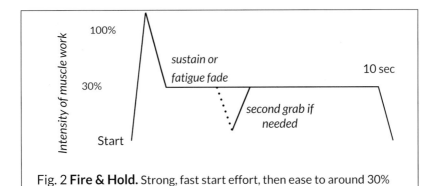

Fig. 2 **Fire & Hold.** Strong, fast start effort, then ease to around 30% for 10 sec. then switch off. If you fatigue, take a second grab.

to recover. Meanwhile, complete your set of ten repetitions using the slow, dimmer-switch holds you mastered in Level One. With training, the number of repetitions to fast-twitch fatigue will increase until you can complete all ten repetitions.

Fire & Relax

The second pattern for Level Two is a pulsing of your pelvic floor muscles on and off. Rapid 'on' followed by rapid and <u>total</u> 'off'. (Fig.3). As you become more explosive in your activation you may inadvertently start sucking in your ab muscles to 'help', especially as you fatigue during a set. One word: don't. If you can only do 10 or 12 reps correctly, your training dose is 'failure plus two': 12 or 14 reps respectively. This will prevent you becoming skilled at

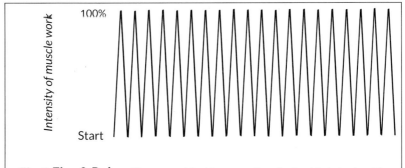

Fig. 3 **Fire & Relax.** Strong and fast turn on, then instant total relax. Then explode again, and totally relax. Repeat until fatigued or up to 20 reps.

doing them incorrectly. A second indicator of fatigue is a slow down of the switching off phase and an early reactivation before total relaxing of the pelvic floor: more of a flutter than a pulse. In this case, slow down, switch off each time, then repeat. You will gradually become as skilful with the 'off' phase as you are with the 'on'. Both phases are equally important for control training.

New Prescription

Let's stay with the 60 repetitions per day but mix it up a bit. You now have three pelvic floor exercise patterns:

1. Slow, prolonged low intensity: Level One
2. Fast and strong with a low intensity hold: Fire & Hold
3. Fast on, fast off and repeat: Fire & Relax

Your daily routine should include all three patterns. I suggest for every Level One rep you complete five reps of the Level Two, for example, do 10 Level Ones, 25 Fire & Holds and 25 Fire & Relax as a minimum daily training dose. You can do more but not less.

Breathing is still important; simply breathe normally during your exercises. And at all other times.

Level Two Video is at craigallingham.com.

Summary of Level Two

» Learn the *Fire and Hold* and use the second grab until you don't need it.

» Learn the *Fire and Relax* ensuring total 'off' between efforts.

» When you can do the exercise while sitting and standing start trying it while walking.

» Tall posture (in sitting or standing) and normal breathing during these patterns of activation.

Level Three - Tighten The Tap

Having mastered the muscle skills to control urine flow, it is time to start building bladder capacity. You have reduced the leaking problem, using fewer or no pads, but you still go to the toilet more frequently than necessary. Perhaps every two or three hours through the day and twice or more through the night. You should aim to do better than that. You need to **'Tighten The Tap'**.

One of the main reasons for urinary frequency is **habit**. It is

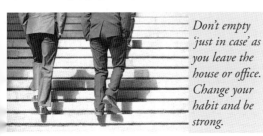

Don't empty 'just in case' as you leave the house or office. Change your habit and be strong.

tempting to empty your bladder whenever you can, when you have the opportunity - just in case. For example, you are leaving the house and take a small leak just in case. Or you are at dinner with friends and you go to the bathroom between courses just in case. This are bad bladder habits.

Another reason is a heightened **sensitivity** to the 'bladder full' signal in your brain. You are finely attuned to this signal in preparation for avoiding mishaps. However, when you are distracted or busy, you find you are going less frequently. Increasing input to the brain will reduce your attention to the 'urgent' bladder signal.

A third reason may be a **decreased bladder capacity**. As a result of repeated premature emptying, your bladder hasn't really regained its full volume. I believe this factor is gravity and/or activity dependent. It is not uncommon for a guy to last four or six hours between bladder emptying overnight, but through the day he feels he needs to empty after two hours or so. When he

31

empties overnight he produces a lot more urine than for the two hour day cycle. This shows his bladder can hold a larger volume when he is horizontal and inactive, but when upright and active the additional pressure increases the signal to empty. The bladder size doesn't change but its emptying cycle is compromised.

Any one, two or three of these factors could be active so it can get complicated. Let's take them one at a time.

Habit

Get over it. I know you are glad to be rid, or almost rid, of the pads, but if this lack of security is part of the 'just in case' emptying, go back to using a pad while trying to extend your time between toilet visits, you can then check the pad to see if there has been any leaking. This way you can manage the risk as you develop better habits and longer filling time.

Once you decide to go to the toilet, it starts a cascade of signals from the brain to prepare the bladder to release and empty. Giving the brain permission to launch may be unstoppable. Try withholding permission: distract yourself with rituals of leaving the house (find the keys, set security, close the drapes) then go out, knowing the pad provides a safe backup, but confident that you won't need it.

> Do you need the night pad, or is it a habit? Two consecutive dry nights - no pad on night three.
> Your next Hero Moment - leaving home pad free.

Posture

Your urinary control muscles partner with those controlling your body posture. They do different things but do them more effectively when they work together. Many men find their continence is worse later in the day. Despite good control all morning they leak more from mid-afternoon. Also, they are less active in the afternoon and evening. Are the inactivity and incontinence related? And if so, which is cause and which is effect?

Research suggests prolonged sitting can lead to a progressive shutting down of our postural muscles as we slump against the 'support' of the chair or sofa. Our pelvic floor muscles are wired with the postural muscle system so they also quieten their resting activity during sustained sitting. Do you sit more because you are tired from the day or are you tired because you sit more? Either way, you may leak more.

My colleague Stuart Baptist noticed these guys do better by working on their posture in sitting and standing, training their anti-gravity muscle systems, improving postural awareness and endurance. He is right. I ask these men to interrupt their sitting every 15 min. and stand as tall as possible for 30 seconds. Also, to avoid sofas, use a more upright chair and focus on sitting as tall as possible. Never fall asleep sitting on a sofa or easy chair, either get up or go lie down. In the car, uptilt the interior mirror to ensure you must sit tall to see where you have been. Combined with the pelvic floor training these strategies can help afternoon leakers considerably.

Sensitivity - Urgency

This feeling of 'I need to go and I need to go **now**' is urinary urge and if accompanied by leaking is *urge incontinence* (UI). It is largely a brain phenomenon rather than a full bladder issue. Knowing the difference is important to avoid mishaps. The best clue is the time since last emptying and a knowledge of what you have had to drink since then. If you reckon the signal is a 'false full', you can try to suppress the urge. If it is a 'true full' signal then you had better go.

Urge Suppression - Brain Training

Ignoring or delaying the urge to empty is an exercise in strong thinking because it is all about the mind. Remember, the bladder is not full, it still has reserve capacity but you are getting a signal to empty which is strong because of your heightened sensitivity. There are a few strategies that may help here:

Distraction. You may already have noticed that when you are busy doing stuff, you 'forget' to go the toilet for a while. And when you finally go there is good pressure and volume. So when you are getting towards your usual time to empty, distract yourself. Get busy and forget about it for as long as you can. Then go.

Long Slow Lifts. You can defuse the urge signal by over-riding it with a different sensation. By increasing the noise arriving at the brain, it pays less attention to each incoming message. The technique is to reproduce the long, slow drawing up that we used in Level One (Fig.1) - the dimmer-switch activation and hold. But don't go anywhere near maximum intensity, the risk of bringing in the ab muscles and squeezing your bladder is best avoided. Aim for, say, 30% intensity at the most and hold it for up to ten seconds, then slowly release. Repeat this four or five times. This is a triple threat strategy: you are immediately distracted by doing the exercise, you are using your pelvic floor muscles to kink the urethra, and you are over-riding the signal to empty.

This technique is particularly useful at night when you try to extend the time between getting up to take (and avoid) a leak. When you rouse and feel the urge (or habit) to go to the bathroom, try four or five long, slow lifts and then roll over and go back to sleep. You may gain ten minutes, an hour or even two hours depending on how early your bladder filling alerts you to empty.

Toe Curls. Seriously - toe curls. Slowly curling the toes of both feet like a fist with your foot and holding at around the 50% intensity (don't go too hard or you will be leaping about with foot cramp). You are correct - the toes have nothing to do with bladder control; however the nerves to the toe-curling muscles share a common origin in the spinal cord and when you activate the toe curlers there is overflow activity for those nerves going to the pelvic floor. This confuses your brain with competing incoming signals.

Five toe curls taking five seconds to curl then five to uncurl (the 5x5x5 program) and then go on with what you were doing. Worth a try. As is rubbing the back of your thigh which also inputs to the same sensory pathway and may suppress your urge.

Bladder Training

You will love this or you will hate it - but at least you get to keep score! In fact, this program involves multiple scoring - you might want to create a chart or a spreadsheet. There is a chart in this book (page 62) that you can copy and complete as you go.

Measuring Instruments

- Kitchen scales - to measure the weight of your full pads. The weight is an indicator of how much urine you have lost, leaked and coughed. The lighter the pad the further your progress. NOTE: Always place the used pad in a plastic bag before weighing. Best if the scales can record in metric units as one gram equates to one millilitre and makes any volume calculations easier. Weigh a fresh pad to establish the dry pad weight to subtract from the used pad total each time.

- Measuring jug - to measure the urine that doesn't end up in the pad. Yep, you pee in the jug* and record the volume each time you empty your bladder. Rinse the jug as you flush the toilet and keep it ready for the next fascinating experiment.

The goal is obviously to have less weight in the pad, more urine in the jug and longer intervals between emptying. All these are indicators of increased bladder capacity and control.

You will also notice on the recording sheet a column for 'Intake' where you record what you drink through the 24 hour cycle. The time and quantity should be logged along with the type of fluid (water, milk, wine, beer, coffee, tea etc). Everything goes on the sheet, because it will relate to the volumes coming out.

---

*It is wise to mark this jug clearly to ensure it doesn't end up back in the kitchen

Method:

For 24 hours (at least) complete the recording sheet. When you go to the toilet pee into the jug, emptying the bladder completely, then read the volume of urine passed. Record this on your chart. Empty the jug into the toilet bowl and rinse the jug under the flush flow. This is now your baseline against which you can monitor improvement. After four to six weeks of the 'Tighten The Tap Program including the exercises, habit control and de-sensitising, complete another 24 hour cycle of measurement and you will have an objective confirmation of what you are experiencing. Sure, you will know whether or not you are improving, but the measurements will confirm how far you have come. Useful data for your medical team too.

Improvement - What will get better?

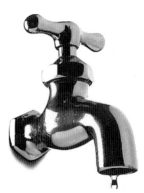

1. Time between emptying - depending on what you have consumed, 4 to 5 hours through the day and one or zero overnight toilet visits.

2. Jug volume - an adult male should pass 400-450 ml per emptying of a full bladder. The urge to empty may start at around 250ml or less for reasons previously mentioned.

3. Pad Weight - zero gain due to zero leak. There may be a slight increase due to absorbing of sweat, but this will be minor.

Summary Level Three - Tighten The Tap

» Bladder training is a learned skill. Persist.

» Tightening the Tap takes effort and mindfulness.

» Dry for 2 nights: stop wearing the pad to bed. Hero time.

» You can't manage what you don't measure.

Level Four - Recovery Tips

Up to now you have been focused on 'Tightening the Tap' to bring your leaking and bladder habits under control. Now it is time to integrate the pelvic floor muscle training and tap tightening with your life, as you are starting to get one back.

Hydration

Some guys try to improve control by reducing their fluid consumption. They figure 'less in = less out'. However this is not a healthy strategy to regain control and reduce leaking. Reduced fluid intake results in highly concentrated urine which irritates your bladder lining prompting it to empty before filling. Frequency and urgency may actually increase! Water is a critical component of our diet and forms the medium within our bodies in which most chemical, regulatory, nutritional and cognitive (thinking) activities occur. Even if your tap is still dripping, you need to keep up your fluid intake.

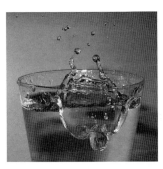

The best fluid is water because it requires no processing by your body before use. Ideally it arrives with no contaminants or elements that need to be filtered or which might slow the absorption. Nor does it contain chemicals that may work against your continence goal. For example, alcohol and caffeine are chemicals that may interfere with your bladder retraining program. You need not swear off them for life, but perhaps for a month or three, then gradually reintroduce them to the level your bladder can tolerate.

One common strategy is to avoid drinking after, say 5pm in the evening in order to reduce the number of times getting up overnight to empty the bladder. Fair enough, better quality of sleep is good for your health. If you adopt this idea, Ensure that you drink a glass of water on your way back to bed after emptying during the night. If you sleep through the night, drink it upon waking as your reserves will be depleted. Not juice, water. Boring? Perhaps, but still the cheapest, fastest way to replenish your body's water table.

Nutrition

What you eat is important for a bunch of reasons, these include:

- » The quality of raw materials used to constantly renew your body structure as cells die and need replacing.
- » For the energy to keep you active.
- » To reduce inflammation in the body.
- » For the effect on your body weight.
- » For taste and shared enjoyment.
- » It will keep you alive.

They are all important but for this program it is your body weight and its effect on your bladder that is critical.

The science of nutrition and weight loss is long, and the myths are even longer. The traditional model of controlling your body weight is anchored in the balance between energy consumed and energy burned. Consume less energy than you expend with activity and you will lose weight. Sadly, the weight loss from removal of a prostate gland is negligible, maybe 60 grams at most, less than 2oz.

The energy-in versus energy-out equation is a simplification that avoids discussing the emotional, psychological and social aspects of food. That doesn't make it any less true, just harder to navigate. Most weight loss diets follow this concept either with reducing quantity of food, replacing high kilojoule (kj) food with lower kj substitutes (protein shakes for example) or some other manipulation of dietary intake. Most programs deliver early results when your enthusiasm is at its best. Staying with it is the greater challenge, especially diets that ban the foods you enjoy or compromise the pleasures of shared dining.

Foods marked as 'low fat' often have added sugar to improve the taste (the flavour-enhancing fat has been removed). High sugar means higher kilojoules to be burned off later or stored as fat.

Sustained weight control is more about long-term behaviour/ attitude change and retraining your preferences than about short-term meal substitutes. This is why it is so very, very challenging.

Losing visceral fat is the key for us guys; this is the fat around our middles that links strongly with health problems including prostate cancer. Other conditions include bowel cancer, high blood pressure, diabetes and auto-immune diseases such as arthritis of the joints, sleep apnoea, tendon degeneration and macular degeneration in the eyes. Reducing added sugar in your diet will help enormously.

Don't become obsessed with your body weight, instead become obsessed with your abdominal girth. The body circumference at the level of your belly button is a great health indicator of how your body is travelling. Keep it below 94cm (37 inches) and you will do all of your vital parts and systems a great favour.

If you need assistance with weight management consult your medical practitioner who may refer you to an accredited nutritionist. This way you receive a balanced, healthy plan and are monitored for any ill effects. Hunger is not an 'ill effect' it is just an effect. You will have to deal with it.

There are myriad exclusion diets, protein-shake meal replacement programs, fad diets, fasting plans and so on in the press and web space. Many of them will achieve weight loss results in the short term by applying the energy equation principle, but they are difficult to sustain and integrate into your lifestyle because they can be so miserable. A future based on deprivation will suck the joy from your life. Find a balance based on 'disciplined indulgence' where you limit your excesses and discover replacements whether they be alternate foods, activities, friends, interests or projects.

Pre-Setting

Using your 'Fast-Switch On' skill just prior to fast-risk activities.

Having trained your fast-twitch fibres to quickly contract and for your slow fibres to then take over to sustain the control (Fire & Hold) all that remains is to take this conscious skill and restore it to a subconscious effect by establishing a new habit.

You already know which activities or movements are most testing for your bladder control. It might be lifting, getting up from a chair, coughing, sneezing, laughing or pretty much any body movement that increases your intra-abdominal pressure and attempts to squeeze urine past your control muscles.

The strategy is to anticipate when you are at risk, or about to be, and to initiate a **Fire & Hold** just prior to lifting, coughing, laughing, etc. If necessary sustain the hold as you carry, push, shout, play the trombone or do other physical stuff.

Anticipate. Every time. It is said that 10,000 correct repetitions turn a habit into a perfected skill so you had better get started. It will take time, there will be setbacks, mis-timings, errors and maybe embarrassments. But none of these is a reason to give up. Quite the reverse - they are your motivation to keep at it.

Examples of pre-setting activities include weight lifting, walking and squats. Consciously activating your pelvic floor muscles just prior to load or holding a sustained low level lift whilst walking will control bladder leakage. This is integrating pelvic floor muscle work with other activities in your life.

When you pre-set, if you feel a small urine leak it is most likely to be a puddle of urine in the urethra below the level of your pelvic floor muscles (after-wee) or you have a slow bladder leak pooling below where your pelvic floor muscles constrict and kink the urethra. When you 'Fire & Hold' the pressure squirts the puddle out. Suggestions for each:

1. Milk residual urine from your urethra after urinating by stroking forward along your perineum and/or do 5 reps of Fire & Relax. Shaking alone won't do it.

2. Revisit Level One for a few weeks. Work on slow, low level holds to reduce slow leaking at rest. And stand/sit tall during urination. If it persists, speak to your medical team.

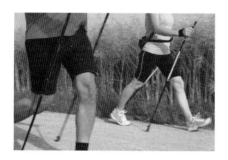

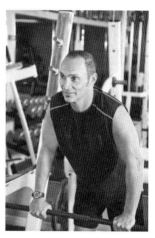

Summary of Level Four

» Water is the drink of choice for bladder training
» Minimise coffee, alcohol and sugary drinks
» Reduce or keep your abdominal girth to 94cm (37") or less
» Practice pre-setting your pelvic floor muscles until it becomes a habit

Level Five - The Masterclass

If you are ready for this level you have done a great job. If you are just reading ahead to see what is coming, or to take some shortcuts - get back to where you were up to. With persistence you may get to this level, but not all guys will make it, nor will all need to. If you have earned it, welcome and let's go.

From the beginning we have been trying to reduce the abdominal muscle overload whilst engaging the pelvic floor muscles to maximise the control and training effect. It is time now to train the floor muscles to work in conjunction with the ab muscles, but not to be overwhelmed by them. This is important, because when you lift correctly at work or in the garden or with grandchildren you will engage your abdominal wall muscles to brace and protect your spine. When this happens you don't want to be worried about whether you will leak a bit under load (because you are probably no longer wearing pads).

Two simple abdominal training exercises are suggested here. One is a strong postural hold and the other involves some movement. Both are important to prepare for the unexpected demands of an active life. I didn't invent these exercises but have used them for many years to good effect. They are also part of my exercise routine.

The Plank

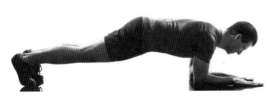

We can use this holding position against gravity to strongly engage the abdominal muscles. Just prior to adopting the position, lift and hold your pelvic floor muscles as you have been training and sustain it for as long as you can in the plank position. If your pelvic floor muscles fatigue and can't be fired again with a second effort, rest from the plank and repeat when able. Starting level is usually five planks with pelvic floor activation for up to 10 seconds each.

If you find the full length exercise too challenging, use the Knee Plank variation: same technique but from your knees.

McGill Curl Up

This fabulous abdominal training exercise is considered by many to be the safest and most effective variation of the traditional curl. You are not using it for ab training, that will be a side benefit. You are using it to sustain a pelvic floor contraction while activating your abdominal muscles by lifting your upper torso.

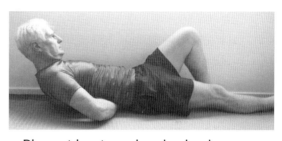

Start flat on your back on a firm surface. Have one leg bent such that the heel is on the floor and level with the opposite knee. Place at least one hand palm down beneath your low back, in the natural hollow. Now engage your pelvic floor muscles at 50% intensity and maintain it as you lift your head and shoulders off the floor. Slowly curl up until your shoulder blades clear the floor. Sustain the pelvic floor activity as you take a few regular breaths in this curl position, then lower your head before finally releasing the pelvic floor muscles. Rest and repeat X 5. This exercise progresses by extending the holding time up to 30 sec or so rather than doing more reps, although you could go up to 10 reps quite safely.

If this exercise strains or pains your neck, cease it and continue with the rest of the program.

43

Your Plan

Begin with the Plank and when you feel confident sustaining a pelvic floor lift with the abdominal muscles working, you can add the McGill Curl Up. You don't need to do these every day - four sessions across a week will provide a good training effect. Remember to breathe while doing both of these exercises. On no account hold your breath during the muscle training.

Squats

There are squats and there are squats. This one is a flat footed squat I call a Butt Squat. Combined with a pelvic floor lift it becomes a Pelvic Floor Squat. The key points are:

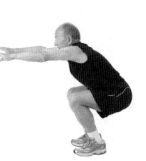

- » Head up and eyes straight ahead (no looking downwards)
- » Both arms extended forwards for balance
- » Low back stays slightly hollowed or flat
- » Your butt pushes backwards keeping your knees behind your toe-line
- » Weight on heels, no lifting them

Just prior to squatting, lift your pelvic floor muscles as you breathe out (Level One) maintaining as you lower to your comfort limit on the squat and then rise again. Relax your pelvic floor briefly, and repeat. If too easy you can add hand weights of up to 4kg.

Once you have mastered the Plank, Curl and Squat with no leaking of urine, you may progress. I suggest you spend at least four months of consistent training on the three exercises described above before attempting the next one.

The Turkish Get Up

Now this exercise is a real cracker and not all of you will get it done. You may have low back, hip, knee or shoulder problems that prevent you performing the movement correctly. Don't force it.

This will test your pelvic floor muscles and bladder control to a level you may never be quite ready for. The Get Up is a total

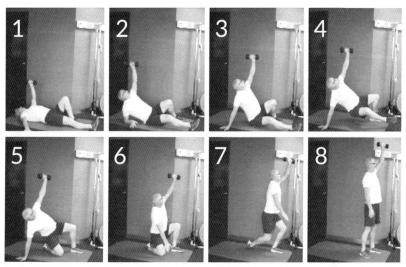

Frame by Frame -The Turkish Get Up

1. Start flat with knee bent on the same side as arm is raised
2. Push through L heel to roll onto right elbow
3. Extend R arm to prop on R hand, drop right shoulder
4. Raise your hips (bridge) so you can pass your R leg beneath the L leg and rest on the R knee
5. Shift your balance over R knee and left leg
6. Rise to standing with head up, eyes locked on the extended arm until upright
7. Keep arm up, relax both shoulders and level your head
8. Pause and reverse to Get Down. Swap arm/leg and repeat.

body exercise emphasising postural control as you get up and down from the floor. The objective is to initiate your pelvic floor engagement just prior to beginning the Get Up and to sustain it during the whole movement. Relax briefly while standing then re-engage for the Get Down. Repeat until you cannot sustain the pelvic floor holds up to a maximum of five to each side.

Start this exercise with no hand weights until you are comfortable with maintaining the extended arm position while locking your gaze on your hand all the way through the movement. Progress to 2kg dumbbell and then maybe 5kg provided you are controlled, safe and both pain and leak free. Heavier weights are not required for pelvic floor muscle training.

There are lots more exercises we could add here, but if you can master these four while maintaining quality pelvic floor muscle control you will be OK for pretty much anything life throws at you.

Videos for the Squat and the Turkish Get Up are at
www.craigallingham.com click on 'MAP Videos & Links'

Summary of Level Five

» Training for 'ordinary' may not be enough.

» Only consider this level if you have no medical or physical conditions that may be aggravated by these more advanced activities. Check with your medical team if unsure.

» Strive for perfect form with total pelvic floor muscle control.

» Combine with healthy living habits for best results.

So Why Don't I Feel Great Yet?

As I have said throughout, not all men will respond equally to this program. There are a range of possible reasons, including the obvious one that this is not the right program for every bloke. You won't know this until you invest time and energy for at least six weeks. At the six week mark you should see improvements that will themselves motivate you to keep going. If not, you may need to consult your health professional and tell him/her what you have been trying. Beyond that, and even if you are getting some results in terms of leaking, urge control, less pad use and longer intervals between emptying, there are many reasons why you may not be feeling great yet. Not all them are physical, so talk openly with yout medical team to allow them to help you.

Turning Exercises into Training

For the exercises to make a long term difference they need to become training. Which means you must do them according to the program - correct technique, repetitions per day, days per week and working to fatigue. If you don't do the exercises you can never claim that the program wasn't effective. You were ineffective, not the program. On the other hand, you may be committed and almost obsessed with the program to the point where it is all you think about - get over it. There are lots of other areas in your life that are more fun than these darned exercises. Invest time and energy in those areas too, your relationships, hobbies, recreations, mates, collections, family history, cleaning out stuff, and so on. The exercises are not the reason you underwent cancer removal surgery - they are just part of the recovery process. Recovery between exercise bouts is also important so don't overdo it.

Healing

Men heal at different rates. Your body has been under attack, not only from the cancer but also from any drugs, radiation therapy and the surgery itself. Your recovery resources have been depleted and it will take time to rebuild. Good nutrition, hydration and positive living will help, but it still takes time. Accept help from within the family and from your mates. It is a sign of strength to accept graciously the help of others, not a sign of weakness. Those offering to help may do so because they otherwise feel helpless and by being of some assistance they also benefit as they see you recover.

Depression

A very common problem when blokes are confronted with their mortality and the realisation they are not invincible. Combine this with the indignity of the diagnostic and treatment process, the withdrawal from work and other social groups, the feelings of embarrassment and shame due to incontinence and loss of masculinity due to erectile dysfunction and it is a wonder any guys get through this without becoming depressed. This is a common response that should resolve as you mentally adjust and physically recover. If not, speak with your medical support team, there is much that can be done to manage depression.

Virility

Not just sexual, but a lack of strength, motivation and enthusiasm for lots of things. This may partly be depression but also a physical weakness due to lack of activity, being sick and recovering from surgery, chemotherapy, radiation therapy or hormone therapy. I hear comments such as, what's the point, it's too damn hard, nobody understands, I'm sick of doctors, I'm not getting anywhere, I wish I hadn't had the operation.

These comments are dangerous, negative self-talk that if not caused by depression will certainly drag you in that direction.

True, you may not yet feel like the man you were just a few months before the diagnosis and treatment, but you are still a man and need to step back and take stock of what is going well for you. For example:

» loyal and supportive partner

» skilled and knowledgeable health practitioners

» mates staying in contact

» you are alive

» your kids and/or grandkids still love you

» your penis mightn't work well, but your hands, legs, back and brain are still fully operative

» you have this great book

» add your own stuff here:

Sex Life

Possibly, your love muscle is now a love slug. But your most important sex organ is still fully functioning, or it can be if you exercise it. This is your brain, or more accurately, your mind. The plumbing may be down and the wiring kaput, but your Fat Controller (apologies to Thomas the Tank Engine) is still looking around and ready to send out orders.

Some guys recover erectile function spontaneously, indicating the surgeon has spared all the nerves and the blood supply to the penis is strong enough to enlarge the organ. I recall my first post-vasectomy erection and the overwhelming feeling of relief that everything was working. Following prostate surgery I imagine the same event must be a million times more exciting given the low expectations.

The penis needs two things to get up. Firstly it needs adequate blood flow to become rigid. It also needs a nerve signal to close the muscular gates in order to trap the blood in the penis. Prostate surgery doesn't interfere with the blood flow, but it can damage (stretch, tear or cut) the nerve supply that controls the gate-keeping muscles. These muscles are not under voluntary control like your biceps or calf muscles. You can't activate an erection voluntarily, except via the mind, where you can see, imagine, hear, dream, read or talk about something that elicits an arousal response leading to an erection. Prostate surgery does not interfere with your brain, but it can mess with your mind. If you have pain, swelling, anger, fear, lack of faith or anything else blocking the mental aspect of arousal, your most powerful sex organ (your brain) is disabled.

Nerves damaged during surgery can heal. If nerves associated with erectile function are stretched or partially torn/cut, they will heal. It may take up to a year or so for the slow-healing nerves to become electrically connected again to allow the mind to engage the penis. Problem is, if you haven't activated the erectile muscles for six months or so, they may not be particularly responsive or not strong enough to trap the blood in the penis. If you have intact wiring but deconditioned muscle, the result is the same - no action.

Penis Life Support

Your penis needs these elements to become erect

» *strong blood flow*
» *connected wiring*
» *elasticity*
» *aroused mind*

It does not need

» *alcohol*
» *fear*
» *distraction*

There may also be a loss of elasticity as the penis has not been engorged for ages. Particularly if you have neglected to manually stretch it lengthwise during recovery (every few days or so). You may not even realise the nerves have recovered because there is no evidence to the contrary. Mind you, not only has the penis not been exercised for the six months, but with everything else going on, the stress, the fatigue and the effort to regain continence, you and your partner probably haven't given much attention to any horizontal folk-dancing. So your mind hasn't really had much exercise in that direction either.

Another factor is blood flow, it must be sufficient to engorge the penis when the gate-keeper muscles close down the exit. If you have poor blood supply to the heart, your heart doesn't work so well. If you have poor blood supply to your calf muscles, you don't walk so well. Poor blood supply to the penis can be as problematic as nerve damage and lack of use. One of the main causes of erectile dysfunction, apart from prostate surgery, is narrowing of the penile arteries due to atherosclerosis (fat plaques in the vessel walls). Similar narrowing of heart arteries leads to a heart attack, in the penis it is a 'hard attack'. Check your blood lipids and cholesterol and pay attention to the results.

Penile Rehabilitation

Your goal is to restore erectile function back to your recent, pre-treatment level of performance. Consider this, following a hip replacement we aim for pain free walking, stair climbing and typical daily activities. We don't aim to return a man to activities he hasn't done for years, such as football or sitting cross legged on the floor. Your recent erectile performance is your realistic goal.

Penile rehab starts before treatment. This is the time for erectile training to ensure your organ is in the best working condition before the cancer is dealt with. Several erections per week for a few weeks beforehand is your goal. If this is already your habit, just keep at it despite your new worries. If you are out of condition you may need some assistance from visual or manual stimulation, pharmacological help and setting aside time.

Following treatment don't focus on intercourse. Penile rehabilitation is about maintaining a healthy penis that is elastic, has good blood supply, pain free, straight and responsive. A healthy penis increases the chance of successful erections and

51

intercourse in the future without the pressure of striving to accomplish penetration or orgasm too early in your recovery. That said, see point one below.

Much can be done to facilitate the return of erectile function after prostate surgery, for example:

1. Don't give up on sex. Even if you don't regain penile hardening there is a lot of sexing still available.

2. Think about it. Talk about it with your partner. Stimulate your mind even if your apparatus is not yet ready. Be cheeky, approachable, fun, resilient and open.

3. Reduce your cholesterol levels, blood lipids (fats) and body weight. Eat smart, drink less alcohol, be more active.

4. Exercise the penis to retain elasticity and engorgement capacity (using manual stretching, medication, vacuum pumps and/or injections). Talk to a men's health doctor or therapist about your options. Eliciting a real or simulated erection at least twice per week should retain elasticity and oxygen flow to the tissues.

Keep this program up for at least twelve months as you wait for nerve recovery. Even if your organ doesn't rise to its previous majesty, by now you will have learnt some new skills and activities that might be a satisfactory alternative.

Your doctor may prescribe medication to facilitate the neuro-chemical pathway resulting in an erection. The most common are Viagra, Cialis and Levitra, collectively labelled PDE-5 inhibitors. Each has a different active ingredient and similar side effects, chiefly headaches, flushing or stomach upset. At their usual dosages they are 'on-demand' helpers meaning you take them when you want an erection in the next few hours. Cialis stays in the body for longer which extends the response time up to eight hours. It also has a low-dose option which is taken daily and allows you to respond at any opportunity. All of the PDE-5 require an additional ingredient to work: arousal. You will need to be stimulated as all these pills are activated by nitric oxide which is produced in the smooth muscle of the penis when aroused. These drugs can take up to six weeks to become effective, so don't give up too early. Men respond differently to each of the PDE-5 drugs, plus you may be taking other medications or have other health conditions that need to be considered. Work with your doctor to ensure your safety and best result. Never try a pill from a mate to see if it works. As if you would.

The use of injections directly into the shaft of the penis to generate erections is not unusual and is far less eye-wateringly painful than most men fear. This is a different drug and does not depend on contextual stimulation (arousal), it just happens with some manual prompting. You will need professional training to master the injection technique, establish your dosage and to learn how to undo a prolonged erection (priapism) which is not only painful but dangerous to your penile health.

The penis pumps create a vacuum in a sealed tube placed over your penis which draws venous blood into your organ. While this provides the physical elongation and girth-stretching for your penis, the blood has only a small amount of oxygen so doesn't help with keeping this aspect of your penis healthy.

Once erectile function returns, through whatever strategy, there is no guarantee it will keep on happening. Particularly if you are undergoing radiation therapy which can undermine erections at some time in the future. Also, the effects of ageing, decreasing aerobic fitness and reduced opportunity for sex may impact on your erectile responsiveness. If this happens, it is worth revisiting the pelvic floor workouts to improve muscular blood flow to your pelvic area. General strength and aerobic fitness is good for all muscle blood flow plus it has been shown to improve the quality of life during and following cancer diagnosis and treatment. Training can also stimulate your immune system to better detect and attack cancer cells perhaps reducing the likelihood of secondary tumours developing.

Orgasm

Achieving ejaculation can occur with or without a full blown erection. While your first orgasm will be a mile-stone in your recovery it can be scary, worrying or just fantastic.

Scary - you may notice some leaking of urine as you arouse your penis. This suggests your continence training is not yet complete. Previously, a muscle at the base (top) of the prostate gland sealed the bladder exit during sexual activity to ensure urine did not escape with the seminal fluid. With limited function of this muscle, you need to be confident your muscle training can cope under this load. Alternatively, you can use a condom to ensure any small urine leakage does not enter your partner. And be sure to empty your bladder beforehand.

Worrying - when you climax it will be 'dry'. Your seminal vesicles and prostate gland were responsible for producing your seminal fluid so without them you will have the sensation of ejaculation without the familiar fluid release. This is your new reality, find something else to worry about.

Fantastic - no urine leaking before, during or after the event and an erection that feels good and gets the job done. With no mess.

Masculinity

You are more than a penis life support system. Your manhood is made up of many aspects and there is no doubt a few of them will take a hit during your diagnosis and treatments. You will be poked, prodded, disrobed, ignored, told to do things, treated like a goose, disrespected, embarrassed, shamed, needy, frequently sad and occasionally bed bound. Not a very blokey time. This is your chance to show personal leadership in the face of adversity, to go boldly showing strength of character and persistence of will.* This is a tough time for blokes unaccustomed to being unwell, being a patient and having other people making decisions on

---

Hear that? It's the theme from Superman. Just for you.

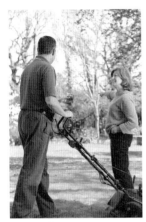

Somedays it may feel like all you do is follow other people's instructions...

their behalf. A very tough time. It may be the first time since your teens that you don't feel in control. Only you can make the mental adjustments to cope with this change. You can take back that feeling of control by learning all you can, by asking key questions and evaluating the answers from doctors and other health providers. Treat this like a project, in which you are both the project as well as the 'project manager'. Apply your understanding of time frames, outcomes, stages, options, extra personnel, out-sourcing, training needs and so on. You can do this.

Mortality

Data indicates that 100% of marriages which don't end in divorce end with the death of one of the partners. We are all going to die. This fact hasn't changed, but has become a lot clearer and poked you in the eye before you were ready. Prostate cancer on its own will not kill you. The prostate gland is not essential for life (they take it out, remember?) but a primary prostate cancer may seed (metastasize) secondary cancers in more vital organs such as the liver, lung or brain. It is also renowned for causing quite painful bone cancers.

Improved surgical techniques are extending the survival prospects for men with prostate cancer. But the surgery is not just to extend your years, it gives you an opportunity to *live* more of your life. Your attitude, support, resources, creativity, nutrition, training, curiosity and persistence will determine the quality of the life you have remaining. None of these strengths was removed with your prostate gland. So *Pad Up, Tuck In and Play On.* And check out the Prostate Playbook (p64).

Barriers to Progress

You

Failure to follow the program. This may be due to lack of application, frustration, inconsistency, pain, boredom, complications, lack of support, or all of the above. It is always your decision as to whether you follow through or not. Be man enough to acknowledge if the fault is yours.

The recovery after prostate treatment is often difficult. You may go through reactions of denial (I'm OK now), anger, despair, blame and resignation. All these are normal but don't get bogged down in any one of them. Push through, try different approaches, talk to other guys, get strength from support groups, share your concerns with mates and family, do stuff you enjoy. Just don't give up.

Pain

Pain in or around the pelvic region is not normal and requires investigation and appropriate treatment. Putting up with it is not heroic, it is lazy or just plain hopeful. Speak with your medical team, tell them exactly what you feel, when and where. If necessary, push to have it investigated. Chronic pelvic pain is not normal and once diagnosed it is usually treatable.

Alcohol

You have undergone major surgery to remove cancer in order to improve your life, so I don't expect you to give up the things you enjoy. However, if they are a barrier to regaining continence you might consider cutting down. Alcohol is definitely one of those.

Many guys tell me they have improved control and decreased pad use during the working week, however on weekends it is not so good. The usual variable is social drinking time. Self control leads to urinary control. Zero acohol beer has improved. Just saying.

Posture

Discussed on page 32 and important enough to remind you again.

Health Status

The better shape you are in the more resources your body can devote to recovery from the surgery. If you are burdened by cardiovascular disease, obesity, diabetes, sleep apnoea, dementia or osteoporosis your immune system and other modulators of recovery will be really under the hammer. Prostate cancer shares risk factors with these other conditions especially with advancing age, so it is common for men to be wrestling with more than one health challenge.

Take care of yourself as best you can in terms of nutrition, alcohol consumption, spending time with mates and doing things that give you a purpose and enjoyment.

Caffeine

Coffee, cola and energy drinks containing caffeine are bladder irritants that can sabotage a continence training program. try de-caff coffee and eradicate the cola/caffeine drinks (empty kilojoules, bladder irritants and calcium leechers). Swap for mineral water or decaffeinated versions of tea or coffee.

Spicy Foods

Some ingredients in spicy foods irritate the bladder. Avoid them until your control improves, then gradually reintroduce them. Pay attention to how you feel regarding urge, frequency and leaking after eating and try to work out what your system reacts to. Then be smart enough to make the adjustments.

Level Six - Cancer Resistant

There are additional strategies that may help your recovery. Some have medical evidence, others are common sense ideas waiting for the evidence. All of these (plus more) are explained fully in THE PROSTATE PLAYBOOK which is your Level Six: building your cancer resistance.

Reduce Inflammation

At any moment there are inflammatory reactions taking place in your body. Inflammation is a normal body process buffered by your immune system but it can get out of balance under stress or extreme load. This can happen if you are unwell, angry, not sleeping, over-working, anxious, depressed, over-exercising. In fact anything that puts your physical or mental life out of balance can affect your general level of inflammation.

Sustained inflammation will depress your immune system at a time when you need it performing strongly as you recover from cancer, surgery, radiation, medication and the associated stress.

There are some simple strategies to try to reduce inflammation that may require new ways of thinking, eating, drinking and living. Some examples from THE PROSTATE PLAYBOOK include -

Vegetables - especially colourful and cruciferous vegetables. All vegetables are good but some are more powerful in terms of their anti-inflammatory effect in your body. Especially when you substitute them for red meat, processed foods, snack foods and milk chocolate.

Visceral Fat (Belly Fat) - this is the preferred area of fat deposition for men. Unfortunately it is also the most dangerous. Being overweight or obese has been found to increase the risk of prostate cancer by 57%[1]. As mentioned previously, fat releases chemicals that exacerbate inflammation in the body. Anything to reduce your girth will help. This may include eating foods you don't prefer and/or doing activities you don't enjoy. If it was easy, we'd all be slim. Info at: *craigallingham.com/girth-control-project/*

Heart-Healthy Diet - replacing a high carbohydrate diet with a Mediterranean style diet rich in vegetables, fruit, oils and nuts will not only protect your coronary arteries but also a range of cancer risks[2]. The preferred oils include olive oil and coconut oil and the nuts should be unsalted or seasoned. Brazil nuts, almonds and macadamia nuts may be the most effective. Eating nuts while drinking beer may undermine the whole concept. Note that the idea is to replace energy intake with more healthy options, not to add them to your current intake.

Perhaps the sneakiest carbohydrate in your current diet is sugar. It is added to many (all?) processed foods and you can find it on the product content labels under 'sugar' and 'energy'. Make a supreme effort to avoid adding it to your foods and choose low sugar/energy alternatives when grocery shopping and dining out. Sugar, especially fructose, is not only inflammatory it offers little nutritional value. It also messes with your liver, kidneys, arteries, blood pressure and brain function. Expect temporary withdrawal symptoms if you exclude it from your diet.

Smoking - Stop now. Absolutely minimise any smoking, active and passive. Identify what it is that smoking does for you and try to find a replacement. You may need help with overcoming

1. Rundle, Jankowski M, Kryvenko O, Tang D, Rybicki B. 2013 Obesity and future prostate cancer risk among men after benign biopsy of the prostate. Cancer Epidmiology, Biomarkers & Prevention, April 23, 2013; doi: 10.1158/1055-9965. EPI-12-0965

2. Richman E, Kenfield S, Chavarro J, Stampfer M, Giovannucci E, Willett W, Chan J. 2013 Fat intake after diagnosis and risk of lethal prostate cancer and all-cause mortality. JAMA Intern Med. 2013;1-8. doi:10.1001/jamainternmed.2013.6536

this addiction in the form of patches, nicotine free e-cigarettes, mentoring, hypnosis and so on. Smoking is not just inflammatory, it can actually set things on fire.

Physical Destressing - the gentle exercise arts of Tai Chi and Yoga are great ways to quiet your busy and anxious mind while working your core postural muscles. You can even add in some pelvic floor muscle training during the session, no one will know. These skills develop posture, muscle endurance, depth of breathing (oxygen is anti-inflammatory) and may help bladder control. They also reduce your stress hormones (cortisol) improving immune function and cancer resistance.

Disciplined Indulgence - I love this concept and try to live my life by its spirit. Indulge in the activities, foods, people and work that you enjoy, but with a personal discipline to ensure you remain balanced and healthy. Think quality not quantity in most things.

Exercise

There is growing evidence that a supervised resistance, aerobic or combined training program is beneficial during and after prostate cancer treatment. Weight (resistance) training helps combat the bone loss due to lowered testosterone and improved fitness can strengthen your immune system response to rogue cells. Seek professional guidance to ensure your program is safe and tailored to your needs. Working in a group where blokes have had a similar experience generally improves your commitment and enjoyment.

Watch the MAP Videos

Find my online videos at www.craigallingham.com or search YouTube for 'prostate recovery map'. They won't win awards, but they might help you improve understanding and application.

The Prostate Playbook - see page 64.

Final Thoughts

You now have the MAP, use it to navigate your recovery before and following prostate treatment.

It is easy to fall into the trap of comparing your recovery progress with other guys, and to despair when hearing of results better than yours. Remember to be sensitive to others if your recovery has been the easier or quicker.

Every man is different. We have different cancers, different health issues, different occupational risk factors, different genetic make up and different surgeons. And no one else has your support crew.

You are not on a journey, or in a battle that has winners and losers. This is simply your new reality. Your priorities have changed and you need new skills. Your individual recovery is yours alone, at times scary, exciting, puzzling, lonely, frustrating and irritating. Deal with what you can and seek help for what you need.

I wish you or your husband, partner, son, father or brother a successful outcome, no matter how you or he measure success. I hope the MAP has been of help or at least some amusement. Gosh knows you could do with something to laugh at.

Now put this book to good use and get on with your program. Don't cheat or take shortcuts, follow the program and give yourself the best chance of success.

Thanks for the opportunity to help,

Craig Allingham

Men's Health Physiotherapist
www.craigallingham.com

48 Hour Bladder Chart - sample entries shown

Date	Time	Jug Vol (ml)	Pad Vol (ml)	Total Vol Out	Fluid Intake
12 Sep	6.05am	350	dry	350	300ml water
	10.45am	240	220g	460	
	11.00am	N/A	N/A	0	250ml coffee
	Totals				

Pad Status: weight or choose from: dry/damp/wet/soaked
Pad Change: Did you change pad? Yes or No (N/A if not using pads)
Fluid Intake – list all consumed